Pharmacology Mnemonics for the Family Nurse Practitioner

Nachole Johnson

Illustrated by Murhiel Caberte

NACHOLE JOHNSON

Disclaimer

Although the author and publisher have made every effort to ensure the information provided in this book were correct at press time, the author and publisher do not assume and hereby disclaim any liability to any party for any loss, damage, or disruption caused by errors or omissions, whether such errors or omissions result from negligence, accident, or any other cause.

This book is not intended as the substitute for the legal advice or consultation of attorneys. The reader should regularly consult an attorney in matters relating to his/her business that may require legal advisement.

ISBN-13: 978-1548378165

ISBN-10: 154837816X

Printed in the United States of America

10 9 8 7 6 5 4 3 2 1

Table of Contents

Chapter 1
Why I Wrote This Book

There's a lot to learn while you are in nurse practitioner school. Because of the time pressure, I really appreciated anything that would help me get through school. I've always been a visual learner, and it is easy for me to pick up information if I draw out pictures or play with words to make learning a complex issue easier. I loved using mnemonics when I was in nursing school, and that continued when I went to graduate school for my Family Nurse Practitioner degree.

I found it was easy for me to remember silly sayings during the test that would remind me of the right answer. Turns out, many other people like mnemonics too! I decided to write a book specifically for the Nurse Practitioner field. Pharmacology Mnemonics for the Nurse Practitioner is a general guide to pharmacology, meaning it will help you no matter your specialty. It is a bit of a cross between what you would expect from a book for nurses and one geared toward physicians.

Use this book as a guide to memorize common concepts and as a refresher for ones you haven't used in a while. Even when you are out of school and in practice, it is sometimes difficult to remember a concept you haven't used since the final exam. This is normal and happens to nurse practitioners and physicians alike. I still use silly mnemonics to remember things like the cranial nerves "**O**n **O**ld **O**lympus **T**owering **T**ops **A** **F**in **A**nd **G**erman **V**iewed **S**ome **H**ops," anyone?

Use this book while you are in school and as a refresher when you finish. I've included extras for Nurse Practitioners like common pharmacological abbreviations, medication classifications, and medication antidotes. Have fun, learn, and enjoy!

Nachole

Chapter 2
Pharmacology Pearls

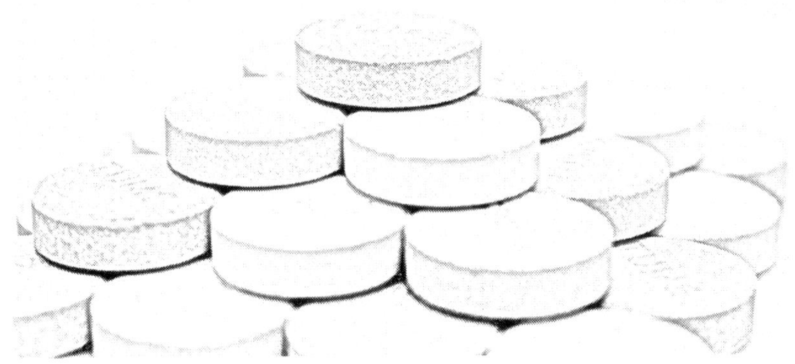

Pharmacology Abbreviations

ā   before

ac   before meals

AD   right ear

AS   left ear

AU   both ears

bid   twice a day

c̄   with

cap capsule

EC enteric-coated

elix elixir

h or hr hour

hs hour of sleep

IM intramuscular

IV intravenous

IVP intravenous push

NG nasogastric

npo nothing by mouth

OD right eye

oint ointment

os mouth

OTC over-the-counter

OS left eye

OU both eyes

$\overline{p}$ after

pc after meals

per by

po by mouth

pr per rectum

prn as needed

q every

q1h every 1 hour

q2h every 2 hours

q3h every 3 hours

q4h every 4 hours

q6h every 6 hours

q8h every 8 hours

qd every day

qh every hour

qid four times a day

$\bar{s}$ without

SL Sublingual

SR sustained release

supp suppository

syr syrup

tab tablet

tid three times a day

Official "Do Not Use" List from JCAHO

Do Not Use	Potential Problem	Use Instead
U, u (unit)	Mistaken for "0" (zero), the number "4" (four) or "cc"	Write "unit"
IU (international unit)	Mistaken for IV (intraveneous) or the number 10 (ten)	Write "International Unit"
Q.D., QD, q.d. qd (daily) Q.O.D., QOD, q.o.d., qod (every other day)	Mistaken for each other Period over the Q mistaken for "I" and the "O" mistaken for "I"	Write "daily" Write "every other day"
Trailing zero (X.0 mg)* Lack of leading zero (.X mg)	Decimal point is missed	Write X mg Write 0.X mg
MS MSO4 and MgSO4	Can mean morphine sulfate or magnesium sulfate Confused for one another	Write "morphine sulfate" Write "magnesium sulfate"

www.jointcommission.org

Drug Administration Routes

Enteral *Oral, Sublingual, Buccal, Rectal* Advantages: convenient, inexpensive, good absorption Disadvantages: Sometimes inefficient, 1st pass effect, irritates gastric mucosa, slow effect, unpleasant taste, can't use if unconscious	**Parenteral** *Intradermal, Subcutaneous, Intramuscular, Intravenous, Intraperitoneal, Intrathecal, Intraarticular, Intra arterial, Intra medullary* Advantages: rapid, can be used for unconscious,. avoid gastric irritation Disadvantages: must maintain asepsis, painful, expensive, possible nerve injury
Topical *Skin, Eye or ear, Nose and Lungs* Advantages: high local concentration without systemic effect Disadvantages: slow onset, local reactions, limited to few drugs, systemic effect with tissue destruction	**Inhalation** *Through nose or mouth* Advantages: rapid onset, large surface area for absorption Disadvantages: most addictive, hard to regulate dosage

Routes of Entry:
Most Rapid Ways Meds/Toxins Enter Body
"Stick it, Sniff it, Suck it, Soak it":
Stick = **I**njection
Sniff = **I**nhalation
Suck = **I**ngestion
Soak = **A**bsorption

Common Medication Classifications and Actions

Antacids- Reduce hydrocholoric acid located in the stomach

Antianemics- Increases the production of red blood cells

Anticholinergics- Decreases oral secretions

Anticoagulants- Prevents the formation of clots

Anticonvulsants- Management of seizures or bipolar disorders

Antidiarrheals- Reduce water in bowels and gastric motility

Antihistamines- Block the release of histamine

Antihypertensives- Decreases blood pressure

Anti-infectives- To get rid of infections

Broncholdilators- Dilates the bronchi and bronchioles

Diuretics- Increase excretion of water/sodium from the body

Laxatives- Loosens stools and increases bowel movements

Miotics- Constricts pupils of the eye

Mydriatics- Dilates the pupils

Narcotics/analgesics- Relieves pain

Pharmacology Suffixes

- **-amil:** calcium channel blockers
- **-caine:** local anesthetics
- **-cycline:** antibiotics
- **-dine:** anti-ulcer agents (H2 histamine blockers)
- **-done:** opioid analgesics
- **-ine:** antidepressants, calcium channel blockers
- **-ide:** oral hypoglycemics
- **-pam:** anti-anxiety agents
- **-oxacin:** broad spectrum antibiotics
- **-micin:** antibiotics
- **-mide:** diuretics
- **-mycin:** antibiotics
- **-nuim:** neuromuscular blockers
- **-olol:** beta blockers
- **-pam:** anti-anxiety agents
- **-pine:** calcium channel blockers
- **-pril:** ace inhibitors
- **-sone:** steroids
- **-statin:** antihyperlipidemics
- **-vir:** anti-virals

- **-xacin:** antibiotics
- **-zide:** diuretics
- **-zine:** antipsychotics

Viral Drugs- "-vir at start, middle or end means virus": ·

Example Drugs:

Abacavir	Norvir
Acyclovir	Oseltamivir
Amprenavir	Penciclovir
Cidofovir	Ritonavir
Denavir	Saquinavir
Efavirenz	Valacyclovir
Indavir	Viracept
Invirase	Viramune
Famvir	Zanamivir
Ganciclovir	Zovirax

Medication Antidotes

Alcohol Withdrawal	Librium
Anticholinergics	Physostigmine
Anticoagulants	Vitamin K, FFP
Asprin	Sodium bicarbonate
Benzodiazepines	Romazicon (Flumazenil)
Beta Blockers	Glucagon
CCB	Calcium, glucagon, insulin
Cholinergic Meds	Atropine, pralidoxime (2-PAM)
Coumadin	Vitamin K
Cyanide	Tydroxycobalamin, sodium thiosulfate
Digoxin	Digiband
Ethylene glycol	Fomepizole,ethanol
Heparin	Protamine Sulfate
Hydrofluoric acid	Calcium Gluconate
Insulin	Glucose
Isoniazid	Deferoxamine
Iron	Deferoxamine
Magnesium Sulfate	Calcium Gluconate
Methanol	Ethanol
Methemoglobin	Methylene blue
Methotrexate	Leucovorin
Opiates	Narcan
Tricyclic antidepressant	Sodium bicarbonate
Tylenol	Mucomyst

Pharmacology Conversions

Volume
1 kiloliter = 1,000 liters = 1 cubic meter
1 liter = 1,000 milliliters = 1,000 cc
1 milliliter = 1 cc
1 fluid ounce = 29.57 milliliters
1 US gallon = 3.785 liters
1 Imperial gallon = 4.546 liters
Weight
1 kilogram = 1,000 grams = 2.2 pounds
1 gram = 1,000 milligrams = 0.035 ounce
1 milligram = 1,000 micrograms = 1/1,000 gram
1 microgram = 10 ^6 grams = 1/1,000 milligram
1 pound = 0.45 kilogram = 16 ounces
1 ounce = 28.35 grams

Additional Conversions:

2.2 lbs = 1 kg

15 gr = 1 g = 1,000 mg

1 gal = 4 qt= 128 oz = 400 mL

1 pt = 16 oz = 480 mL

2 Tbsp = 1 oz = 8 dr = 30 mL

15 gtt = 15 minum = 1 mL= 1 cc

1 lb = 16 oz

1 gr = 65 mg

1 qt = 2 pt

1 L = 1,000 mL

1 cup = 8 oz = 240 mL

1 tsp= 60 gtt 1 dr = 4 mL

1 gtt = 1 minim

1 oz = 30 g

1 mg = 1,000 mcg

Therapeutic dosage: toxicity values for most commonly monitored medications

"The magic 2s":

Digitalis (.5-1.5) Toxicity = 2.

Lithium (.6-1.2) Toxicity = 2.

Theophylline (10-20) Toxicity = 20.

Dilantin (10-20) Toxicity = 20.

APAP (1-30) Toxicity = 200.

Chapter 3
Cardiology

ACE inhibitor side effects (CAPTOPRIL)

- **C**ough
- **A**ngioedema
- **P**roteinuria
- **T**aste disturbance/ **T**eratogenic in 1st trimester
- **O**ther (fatigue, headache)
- **P**otassium increased
- **R**enal impairment
- **I**tch
- **L**ow BP (1st dose)

Alternative - **CRAP PILOT**

C ough
R enal impairment
A naphylaxis
P alpitations

P otassium elevated
I mpotence
L eukocytosis
O rthostatic hypotension
T aste

Beta blockers: **B1 selective vs. B1-B2 non-selective**
A through N: B1 selective: Acebutalol, Atenolol, Esmolol, Metoprolol.
O through Z: B1, B2 non-selective: Pindolol, Propanalol, Timolol.

Beta-1 vs. Beta-2 receptor location

"You have 1 heart and 2 lungs":

Beta-1 acts primarily on heart.

Beta-2 primarily on lungs.

Beta 1 selective blockers

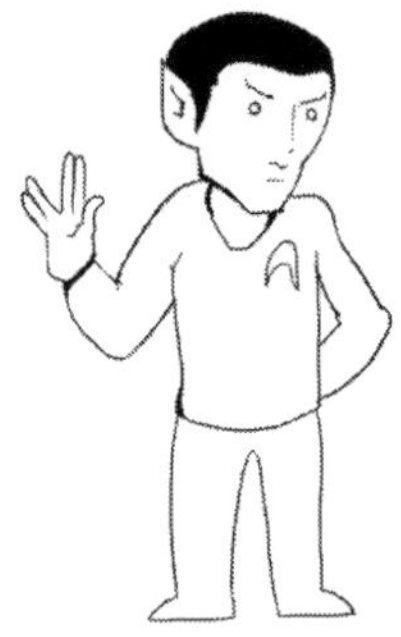

"BEAM me up, Scotty!"

Beta 1 blockers:

Esmolol

Atenolol

Metropolol

Beta-blockers:

Nonselective Beta-blockers:
"Tim Pinches His Nasal Problem"
(because he has a runny nose...):

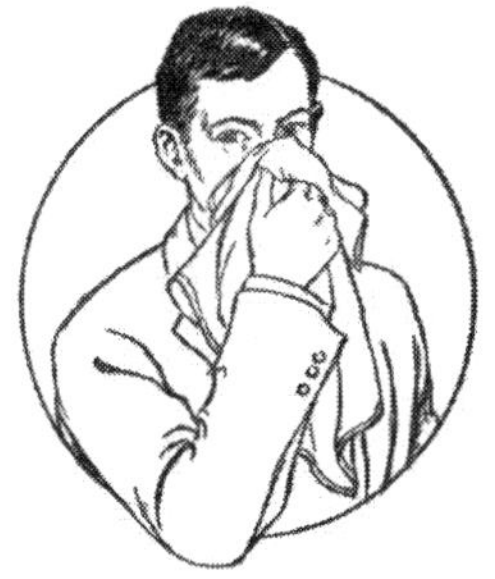

Timolol

Pindolol

Hismolol

Naldolol

Propranolol

Beta-blockers: Side effects "BBC Loses Viewers In Rochedale":

BBC

Bradycardia

Bronchoconstriction

Claudication

Lipids

Vivid dreams & nightmares

Inotropic action

Reduced sensitivity to hypoglycemia

Ca++ Channel Blockers: Uses- CA++ MASH:

Cerebral vasospasm/ **C**HF
Angina
Migraines
Atrial flutter, fibrillation
Supraventricular tachycardia
Hypertension

Alternatively: "CHASM":

Cerebral vasospasm / **C**HF
Hypertension
Angina / **A**trial flutter, fibrillation
Supraventricular tachyarrhythmia
Migraines

Antiarrhythmic: Classification

I to IV ***MBA College***

In order of class I to IV:

Membrane stabilizers (class I)
Beta blockers (class II)
Action potential widening agents (class III)
Calcium channel blockers (class IV)

Amiodarone: Action, Side Effects 6 P's:
P rolongs action potential duration
P hotosensitivity
P igmentation of skin
P eripheral neuropathy
P ulmonary alveolitis and fibrosis
P eripheral conversion of T4 to T3 is inhibited -> hypothyroidism

Direct sympathomimetic catecholamines DINED:

D	I	N	E	D
O	S	O	P	O
P	O	R	I	B
A	P	E	N	U
M	R	P	E	T
I	O	I	P	A
N	T	N	H	M
E	E	E	R	I
	R	P	I	N
	E	H	N	E
	N	R	E	
	O	I		
	L	N		
		E		

Atrial arrhythmias "ABCDE"

A	B	C	D	E
NTICOAGULANTS	ETA BLOCKERS	ALCIUM CHANNEL BLOCKERS	IGOXIN	LECTROCARDIOVERSION

Chapter 4
Pulmonary

Pulmonary Infiltrations Inducing Drugs
"Go BAN Me!"

Gold
Bleomycin/ **B**usulfan/ **B**iCNU **A**miodarone/ **A**cyclovir/ **A**zathioprine **N**itrofurantoin
Melphalan/**Me**thotrexate/**Me**thysergide

Antibiotics for TB

STRIPE:

ST	**R**	**I**	**P**	**E**
R	I	S	Y	T
E	F	O	R	H
P	A	N	A	A
T	M	I	Z	M
O	P	A	I	B
M	I	Z	N	U
Y	C	I	A	T
C	I	D	M	O
I	N		I	L
N			D	
			E	

Alternatively, **RESPI**ration
Rifampicin
Ethambutol
Streptomycin
Pyrazinamide
Isoniazid

Asthma Drugs: Leukotriene Inhibitor Action

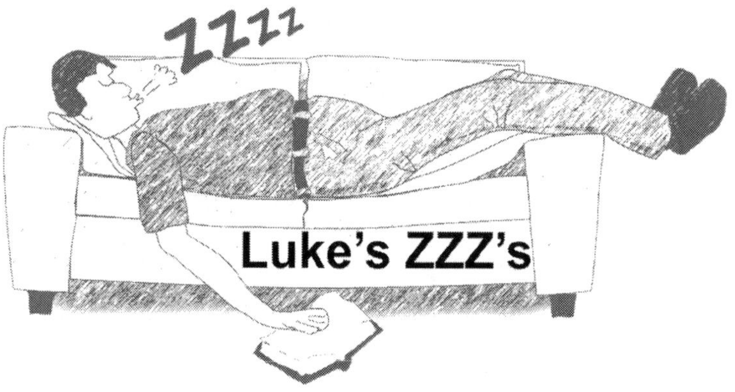

zAfirlukast: Antagonist of lipoxygenase
zIlueton: Inhibitor of LT receptor

Zafirlukast, Montelukast, Cinalukast: Mechanism & Usage

"Zafir-**luk**-ast, Monte-**luk**-ast, Cina-**luk**-ast": Anti-**Leuk**otrienes for Asthma.

Clinical pearl: Zafirlukast antagonizes leukotriene-4.

Medicines for Asthma

A	gonist of beta receptors and Antagonist of leukotriene
S	teroids
T	heophylline – relaxes bronchial muscles
H	istamine antagonist as prophylactic
M	ucolytics – acetylcysteine (Fluimucil)
A	ntibiotics

Ipr*Atropi*um action: ***Atropine*** is buried in the middle, so it behaves like Atropine.

Respiratory depression inducing drugs "STOP breathing":

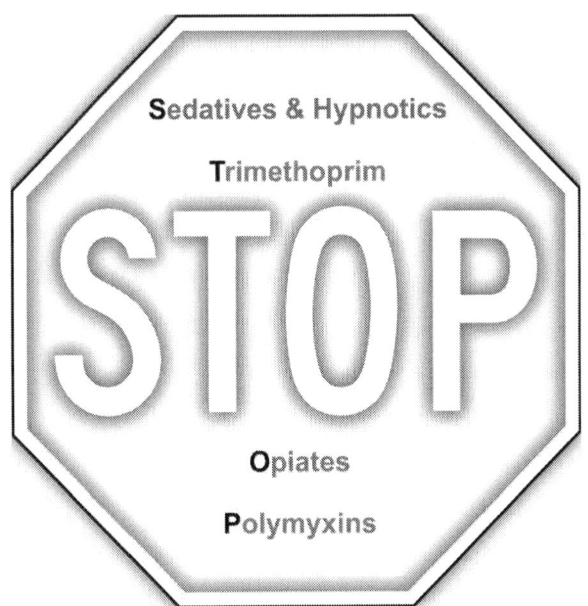

Non-Cardiac Causes of Pulmonary Edema: PONS

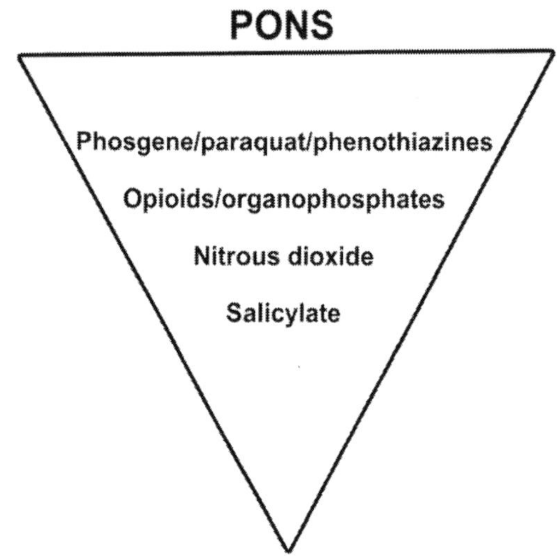

Pulmonary edema "MAD DOG"

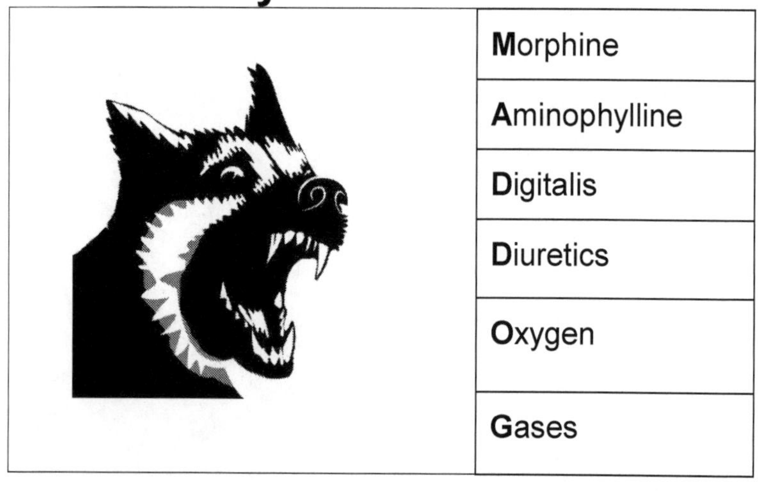

Morphine
Aminophylline
Digitalis
Diuretics
Oxygen
Gases

Chapter 5
Antibiotics/Antivirals

Sulfonamide: Major Side Effects....SSSS

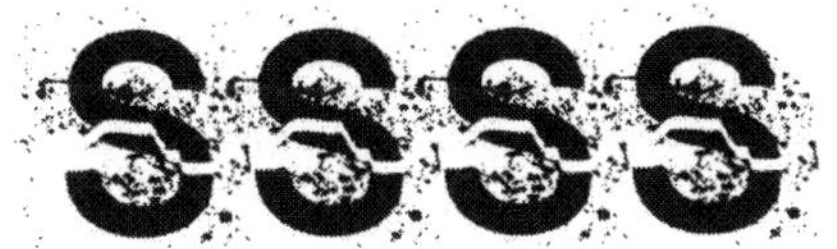

Steven-Johnson syndrome
Skin rash
Solubility low (causes crystalluria)
Serum albumin displaced (Causes newborn kernicterus and potentiation of other serum albumin-binders like warfarin)

Quinolones [and Fluoroquinolones]: mechanism
"Topple the Queen": 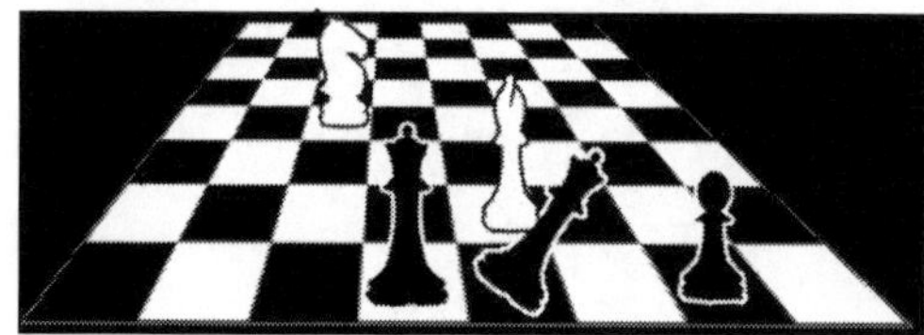 Quinolone interferes with Topoisomerase II.

Nitrofurantoin: Major Side Effects

Nitro**F**ur**A**ntoin:

Neuropathy (peripheral neuropathy)

Fibrosis (pulmonary fibrosis)

Anemia (hemolytic anemia)

Antibiotics Contraindicated During Pregnancy MCAT:

MY MAMA IS A DOCTOR.
MY DADDY IS A DOCTOR.
I AM GOING TO BE A ETERNAL MED STUDENT.
MCAT

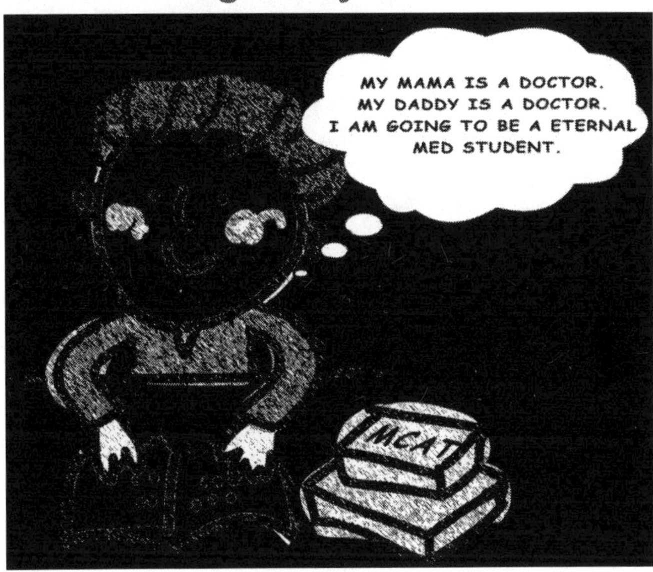

Metronidazole
Chloramphenicol
Aminoglycoside
Tetracycline

Tetracycline: Teratogenicity

TEtracycline is a **TE**ratogen that causes staining of **TE**eth in the newborn.

Vancomycin - "A Red Van Drove Into The Wall"

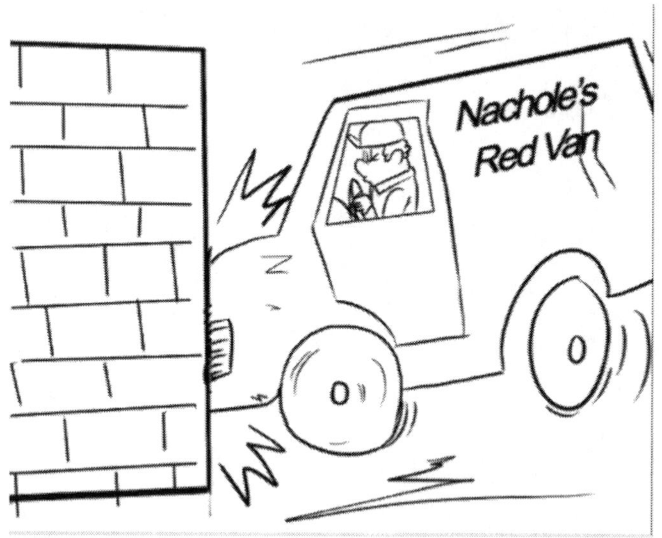

Antihistamines (prevents red man syndrome)
Red man syndrome
Vancomycin
DAla DAla (terminal end of pentapeptide)
Inhibitor
Thrombophlebitis
Wall (cell wall)

Amphotericin Toxicities:
AMPHOTERICIN B

Anemia
Muscle spasms
Phlebitis
Headaches/**H**ypotension/**H**ypokalemia
Other reactions (leukopenia, Increased LFT's)
Thrombocytopenia
Emesis/**E**ncephalopathy
Respiratory stridor
Increased temperature (fever)
Chills
Immediate hypersensitivity (anaphylaxis)
Nephrotoxicity
Bronchospasm

Anti An**X**iety = Bu**X**pirone
Bu**PROPER**ion = **PROPER** habits (no smoking)
It's used for smoking *cessation*.

The Use Of Propranolol
For PERFORMANCE ANXIETY.

Take pr**OPRA-**nolol if you wanna talk to **OPRA**h!!!

Propranolol is the beta-blocker with the strongest sedation effect. Just thinking of talking to Oprah can cause migraines, essential tremors and arrhythmias (the other 3 uses of the drug).

Delirium-Causing Drugs
ACUTE CHANGE IN MS:

Antibiotics (biaxin, penicillin, ciprofloxacin)
Cardiac drugs (digoxin, lidocaine)
Urinary incontinence drugs (anticholinergics)
Theophylline
Ethanol

Corticosteroids
H2 blockers
Antiparkinsonian drugs
Narcotics (esp. mepridine)
Geriatric psychiatric drugs
ENT drugs

Insomnia drugs
NSAIDs (e.g. indomethacin, naproxen)

Muscle relaxants
Seizure medicines

Tricyclic Antidepressants: Meds Worth Knowing

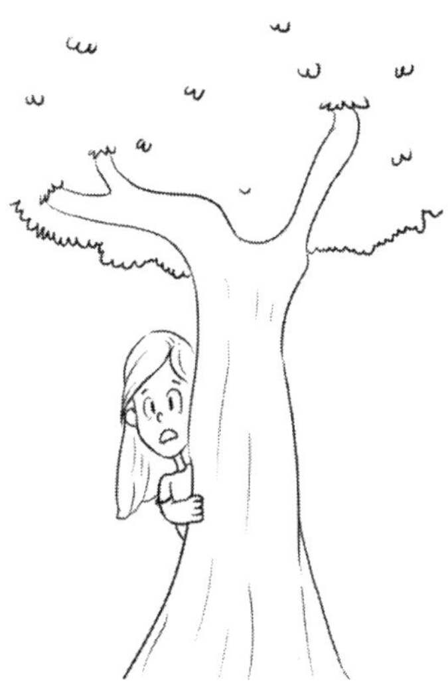

"I have to hide, the CIA is after me":
Clomipramine **I**mipramine **A**mitriptyline

· The next 3 worth knowing,
"The DND is also after me":
Desipramine **N**ortriptyline **D**oxepin

Serotonin Syndrome: Components Causes HARM:

Hyperthermia,
Autonomic Instability (delirium)
Rigidity
Myoclonus

SSRIs: Side Effects SSRI:

Serotonin syndrome
Stimulate CNS
Reproductive dysfunction in male
Insomnia

Depression: 5 Drugs Causing It: PROMS

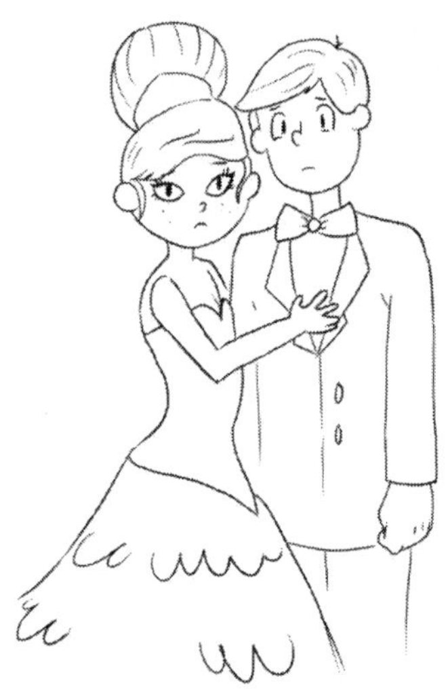

PROPRANOLOL
RESERPINE
ORAL CONTRACEPTIVES
METHYLDOPA
STEROIDS

Benzodiazapines

Benzodiazapines: Those not metabolized by the liver (safe to use in liver failure)

LOT: **L**orazepam **O**xazepam **T**emazepam

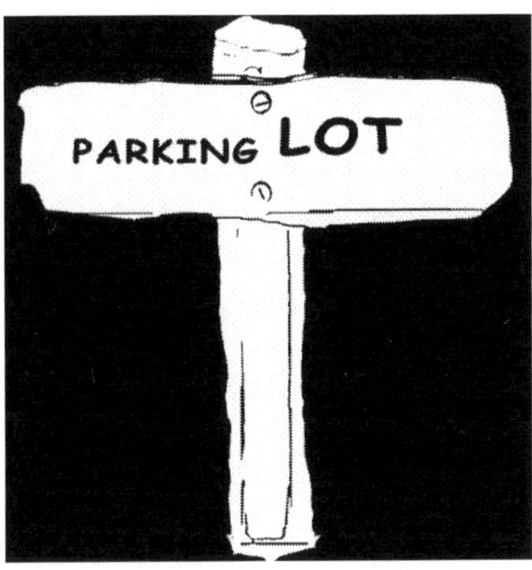

Benzodiazepines: Actions

"Ben **SCAM**s Pam into seduction not by brain but, by muscle":

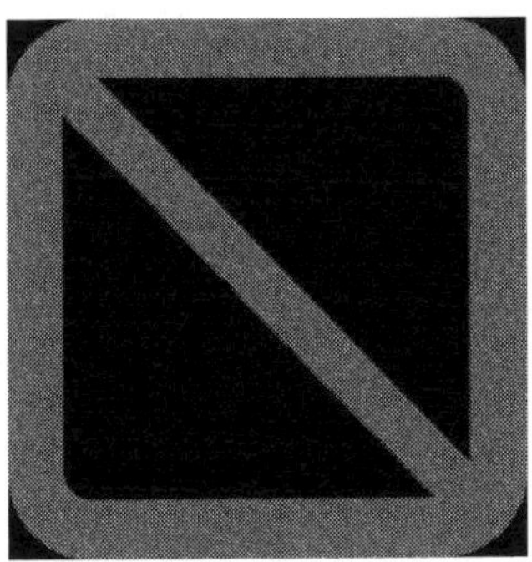

Sedation
anti-**C**onvulsant
anti-**A**nxiety
Muscle relaxant

Not by brain: No antipsychotic activity

Benzodiazepines: Drugs Which Decrease Their Metabolism

"I'm Overly Calm":

Isoniazid

Oral contraceptive pills

Cimetidine

These drugs increase the calming effect of BZDs by retarding metabolism.

Benzodiazepines: Antidote "Ben is off with the Flu":

Benzodiazepine effects off with **Flu**mazenil.

MAOIs: Indications MAOI'S:

Melancholic [classic name for atypical depression]
Anxiety
Obesity disorders [anorexia, bulimia]
Imagined illnesses [hypochondria]
Social phobias
* Listed in decreasing order of importance.

· Note **MAOI** is inside **M**el**A**nch**O****l**ic

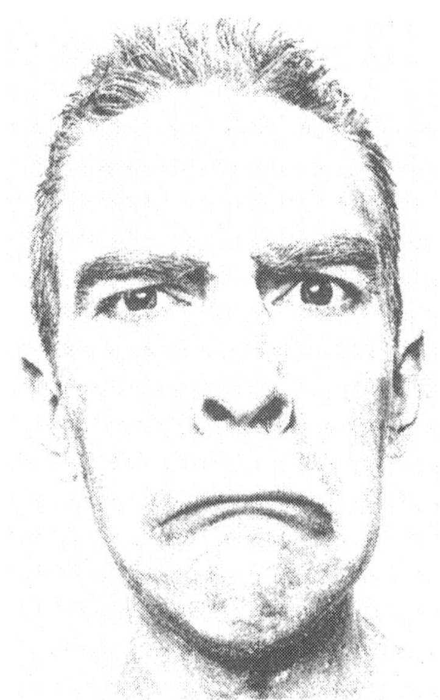

My name is Mel Ancholic.

Monoamine Oxidase Inhibitors:

Members "**PIT** of despair":

Phenelzine

Isocarboxazid

Tranylcypromine

A **PIT** of despair, since MAOIs treat depression

Lithium: Side Effects LITH:

Leukocytosis

Insipidus [diabetes insipidus, tied to polyuria]

Tremor/ Teratogenesis

Hypothyroidism

Chapter 6
Pain

Beneficial Effects Of Inhibition of Prostaglandin

Synthesis i.e. Acetaminophen And NSAIDS (5 A's)

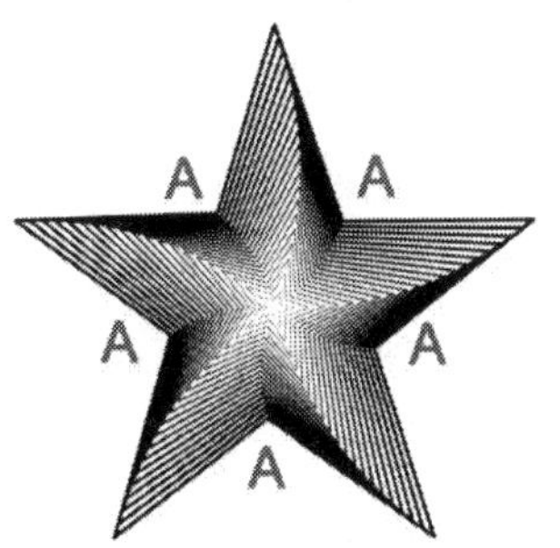

Analgesia
Antipyretic
Anti-inflammatory
Antithrombotic
Arteriosus

(NSAIDs for closure of patent ductus arteriosus)

NSAID Contraindications

Nursing and pregnancy
Serious bleeding
Allergy/**A**sthma/**A**ngioedema
Impaired renal function
Drug (anticoagulant)

Names of Common NSAIDS: CAIN

Celebrex
Asprin
Indomethicin/**I**buprofen
Naproxen

Alternatively, **NSAIDS**

Naproxen
Salicylates
Advil
Ibuprofen
Diclofenac
Sulindac

Narcotics: Side Effects

"SCRAM If You See A Drug Dealer":

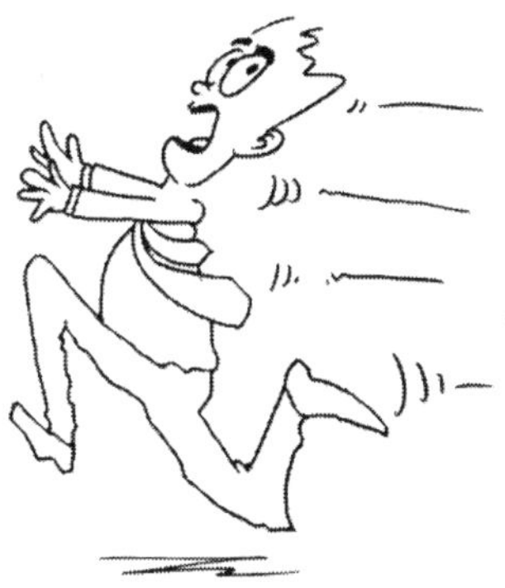

Synergistic CNS depression with other drugs
Constipation
Respiratory depression
Addiction
Miosis

Morphine: Effects MORPHINES:

Miosis
Orthostatic hypotension
Respiratory depression
Pain suppression
Histamine release/ **H**ormonal alterations
Increased ICP
Nausea
Euphoria
Sedation

Morphine Side-Effects: MORPHINE:

Miosis
Out of it (sedation)
Respiratory depression
Pneumonia (aspiration)
Hypotension
Infrequency (constipation, urinary retention)
Nausea
Emesis

Opioids: μ-Receptor Effects "MD CARES":

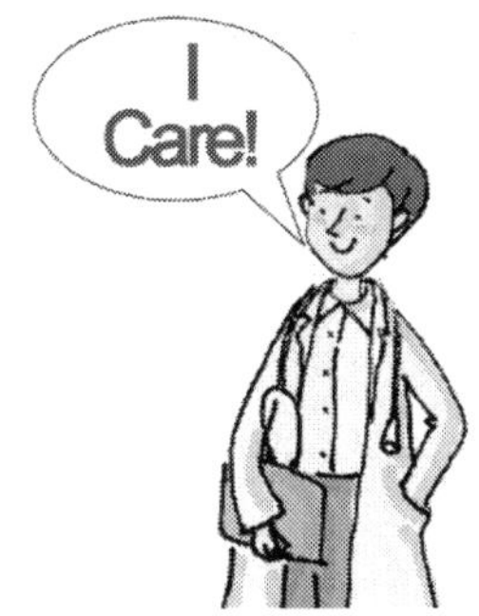

Miosis
Dependency

Constipation
Analgesics
Respiratory depression
Euphoria
Sedation

Opioids: Effects BAD AMERICANS:

Bradycardia & hypotension
Anorexia
Diminished pupillary size

Analgesics
Miosis
Euphoria
Respiratory depression
Increased smooth muscle activity (biliary tract constriction)
Constipation
Ameliorate cough reflex
Nausea and vomiting
Sedation

Narcotic Antagonists

The **N**arcotic **A**ntagonists are **NA**loxone and **NA**ltrexone.

They treat narcotic overdose.

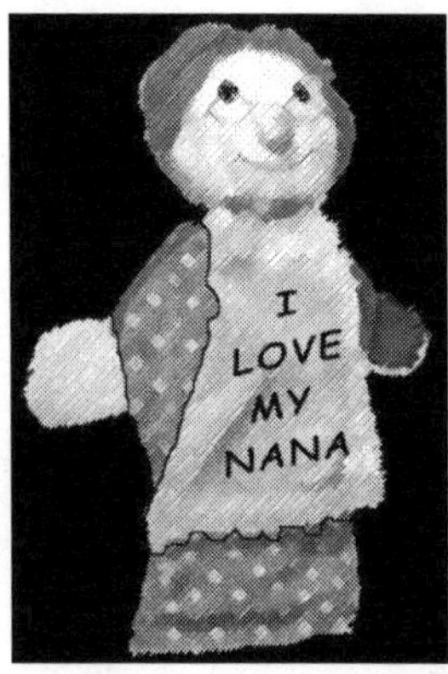

Morphine: Effects At mu-Receptor PEAR:

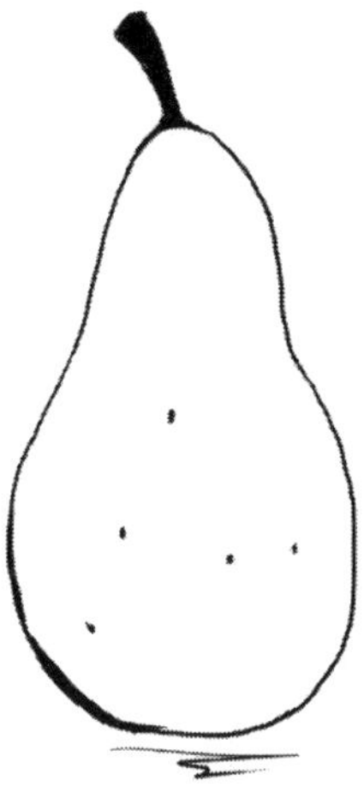

Physical dependence
Euphoria
Analgesia
Respiratory depression

Aspirin: Side Effects ASPIRIN:

Asthma
Salicyalism
Peptic ulcer disease/ **P**hosphorylation-oxidation uncoupling/ **P**PH/ **P**latelet disaggregation/ **P**remature closure of PDA
Intestinal blood loss
Reye's syndrome
Idiosyncrasy
Noise (tinnitus)

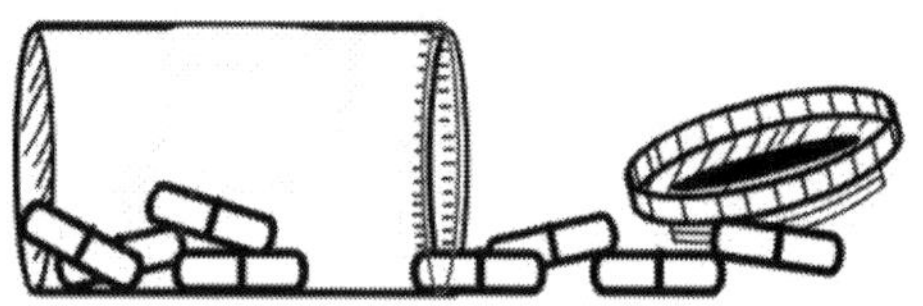

Chapter 7
Endocrine/Immunology

Side Effects Of Systemic Corticosteroids (CORTICOSTEROIDS)

Cushing's syndrome
Osteoporosis
Retardation of growth
Thin skin, easy bruising
Immunosuppression
Cataracts and glaucoma
Oedema
Suppression of HPA axis
Teratogenic
Emotional disturbance
Rise in BP
Obesity (truncal)
Increased hair growth (hirsutism)
Diabetes mellitus
Striae

Steroid Side Effects CUSHINGOID:

Cataracts
Ulcers
Skin: striae, thinning, bruising
Hypertension/ **H**irsutism/ **H**yperglycemia
Infections
Necrosis: avascular necrosis of the femoral head
Glycosuria
Osteoporosis, **O**besity
Immunosuppression
Diabetes

Steroids (6 S's)

Sugar (hyperglycemia)
Soggy bones (causes osteoporosis)
Sick (decreased immunity)
Sad (depression)
Salt (water and salt retention)
Sex (decreased libido)

Steroids: Side Effects BECLOMETHASONE:

Buffalo hump
Easy bruising
Cataracts
Larger appetite
Obesity
Moon face
Euphoria
Thin arms & legs
Hypertension/ **H**yperglycemia
Avascular necrosis of femoral head
Skin thinning
Osteoporosis
Negative nitrogen balance
Emotional liability

Drugs to Use in Rheumatoid Arthritis: MS. AHILA

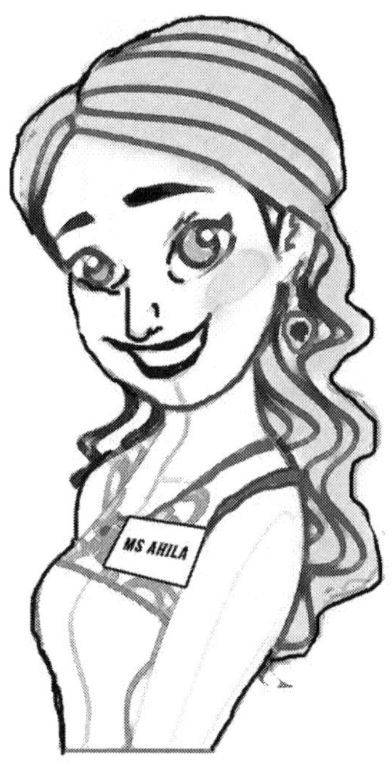

M - Methotrexate
S - Sulfsalazine

A - Adalimumab
H - Hydroxychloroquine
I - Infliximab
L - Leflunomide
A - Abatacept

Busulfan: Features ABCDEF:

Alkylating agent
Bone marrow suppression s/e
CML indication
Dark skin (hyperpigmentation) s/e
Endrocrine insufficiency (adrenal) s/e
Fibrosis (pulmonary) s/e

Antirheumatic Agents (Disease Modifying):

CHAMP:

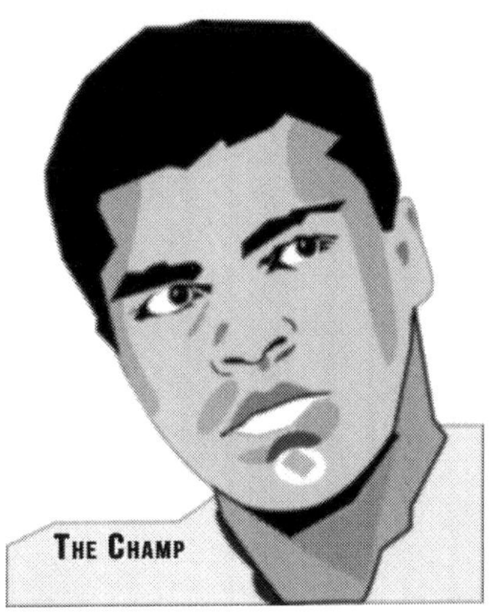

Cyclophosphamide
Hydroxycloroquine and choloroquinine
Auranofin and other gold compounds
Methotrexate
Penicillamine

Auranofin, Aurothioglucose: Category And Indication

Aurum is Latin for "gold" (gold's chemical symbol is Au).

Generic **Aur**- drugs (**Aur**anofin, **Aur**othioglucose) are gold compounds.

Gold's indication is rheumatoid arthritis,
***AUR- A**cts **U**pon **R**heumatoid.*

Enzyme Inhibitors: “SICKFACES.COM

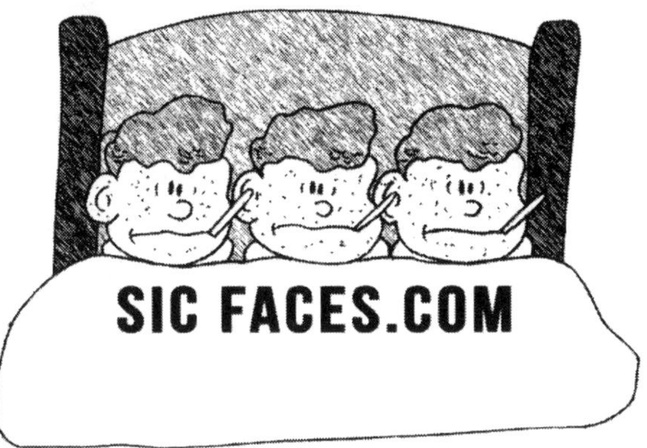

Sodium valproate
Isoniazid
Cimetidine
Fluoxetine
Alcohol
Erythromycin and clarithromycin
Sulphonamides
Ciprofloxacin
Omeprazole
Metronidazole

Lupus: Drugs Inducing It.

HIP:

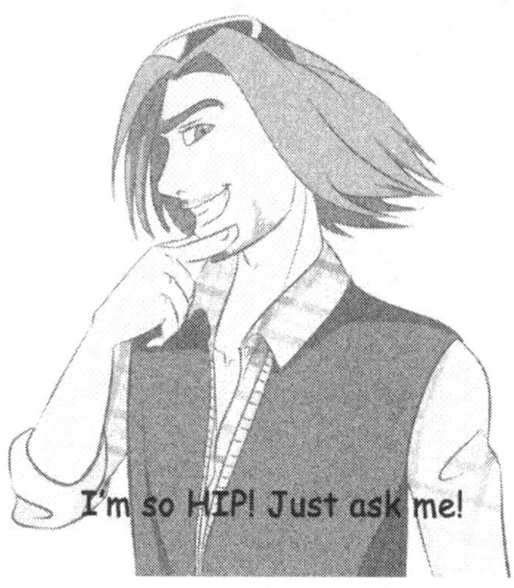

Hydralazine
INH
Procainamide

Chapter 8
GI/Liver

Zero Order Kinetics Drugs (most common ones) "PEAZ (sounds like pees) out a constant amount":

Phenytoin
Ethanol
Aspirin
Zero order

Someone that pees out a constant amount describes zero order kinetics (always the same amount out).

Hepatic Necrosis: Drugs Causing Focal To Massive Necrosis

"Very Angry Hepatocytes":

Valproic acid
Acetaminophen
Halothane

Principles of management in toxicology

RESS

Reduce absorption
Enhance elimination
Specific antidote
Supportive treatment

8 A's for Hepatotoxic Drugs

Anti-tuberculosis
Anticonvulsant
Sodium luminal
Gabapentin
Phenytoin
Tegretol
Anticancer
Aspirin
Alcohol
Antifamily (contraceptive pills)
Acetaminophen
Afatoxins

Inhibitors of p450:

Inhibitors Stop Cute Kids from Eating Grapefruit.

INH
Sulfonamides
Cimetidine
Ketoconazole
Erythromycin
Grapefruit juice

IC(see) KEGS (going down)

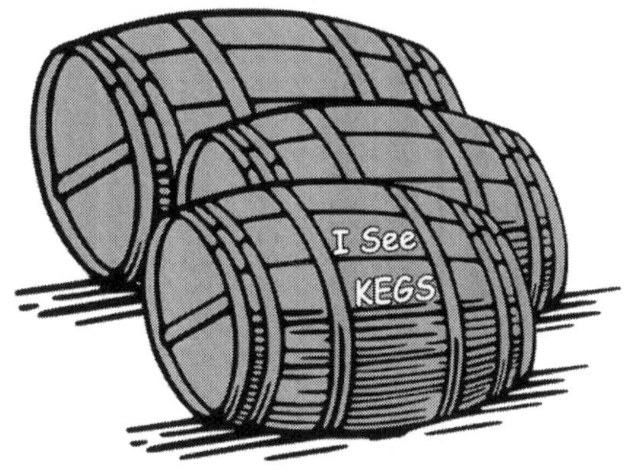

INH
Cimetidine

Ketoconazole
Erythromycin
Grapefruit
Sulfonamides

Chapter 9
GU/Reproductive

Diuretics:

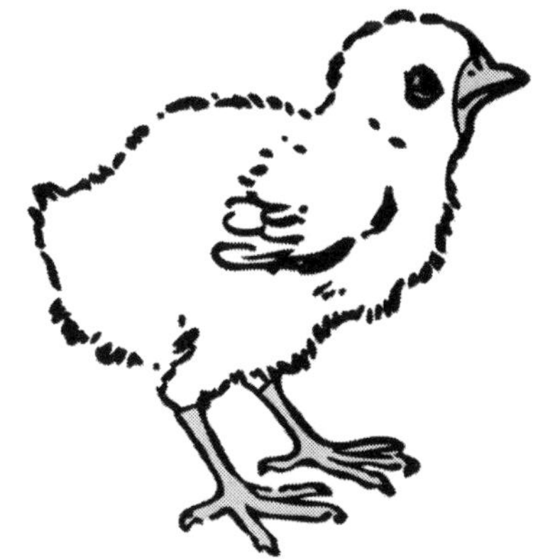

Thiazides Indications: "CHIC"

Congestive Heart failure
Hypertension
Insipidus
Calcium calculi

Osmotic Diuretics: Members GUM:

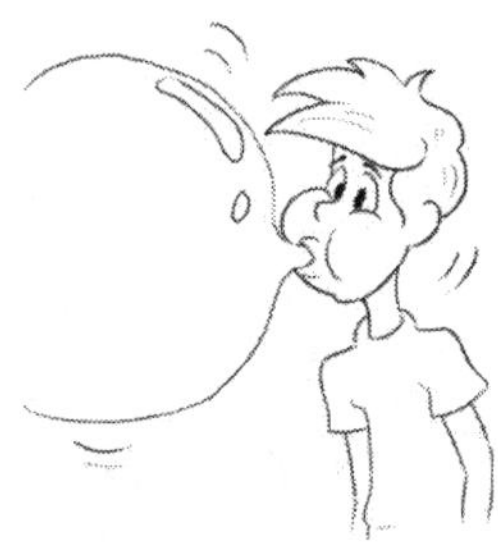

Glycerol
Urea
Mannitol

Teratogenic Drugs "W/ TERATOgenic":

Warfarin
Thalidomide
Epileptic drugs: phenytoin, valproate, carbamazepine
Retinoid
ACE inhibitor
Third element: lithium
OCP and other hormones (e.g. danazol)

Gynecomastia-Causing Drugs DISCO:

D	**I**	**S**	**C**	**O**
i	s	p	i	e
g	o	i	m	s
o	n	r	e	t
x	i	o	t	r
i	a	n	i	o
n	z	o	d	g
	i	l	i	e
	d	a	n	n
		c	e	s
		t		
		o		
		n		
		e		

Alternative,

Gynecomastia Causing Drugs - DISCO 2MTV

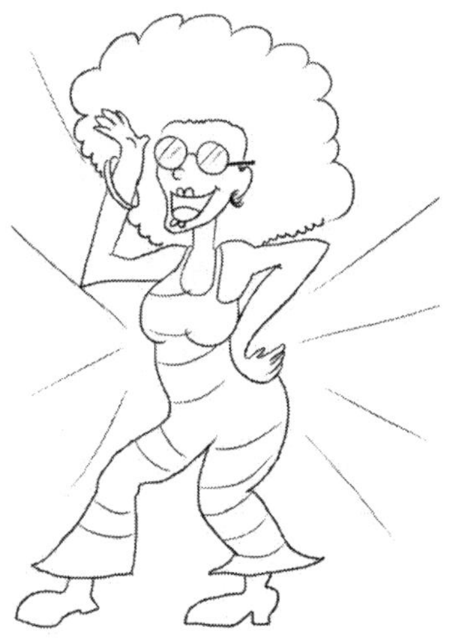

Digoxin
Isoniazid
Spironolactone
Cimetidine
Oestrogens

Methyldopa
Metronidazole
TriCyclic Antidepressants
Verapamil

Sex Hormone Drugs: Male "Feminine Males Need Testosterone":

Fluoxymesterone
Methyltestosterone
Nandrolone
Testosterone

Teratogenic Drugs: Major Non-Antibiotics TAP CAP:

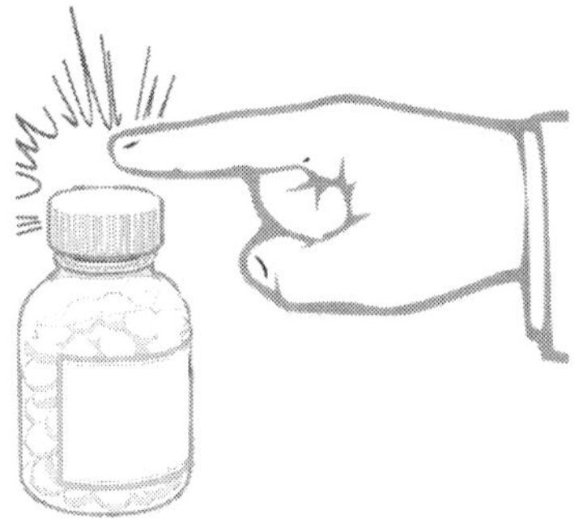

Thalidomide **A**ndrogens **P**rogestins
Corticosteroids **A**spirin & indomethacin **P**henytoin

Don't Use 'Safe CT' in Pregnancy

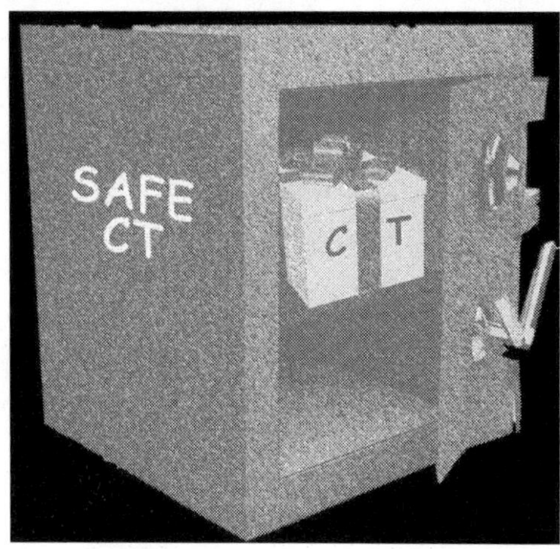

Sulfonamide
Aminoglycoside
Flouroquinolones
Erythromycin

Clarithromycin
Tetracycline

Drugs Causing Erectile Dysfunction

STOP Erection

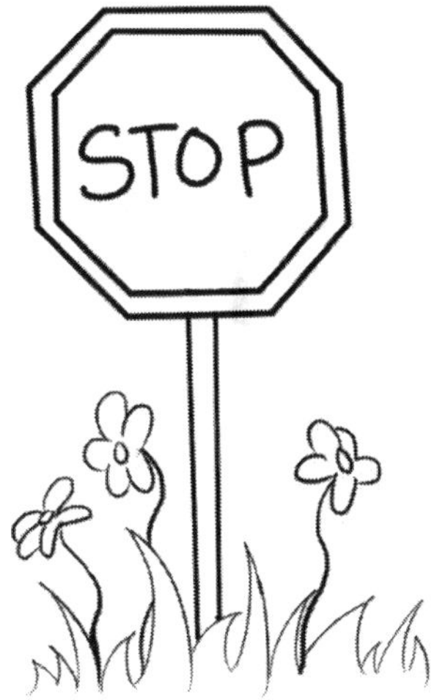

SSRI (fluoxetine)
Thioridazone
Methlyd**O**pa
Propranalol

Uterine Relaxants "It's Not My Time"

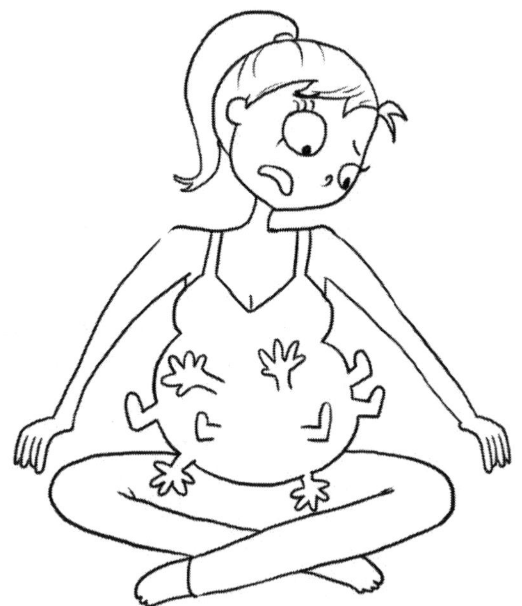

Indomethecin
Nifedipine
Magnesium
Terbutaune

Chapter 10
Hematology

Drugs That Potentiate Warfarin (O DEVICES)

- **O**meprazole
- **D**isulfiram
- **E**rythromycin
- **V**alproate
- **I**soniazid
- **C**iprofloxacin and **C**imetidine
- **E**thanol (acutely)
- **S**ulphonamides

Drugs That Decrease The Effectiveness Of Warfarin (PC BRAS)

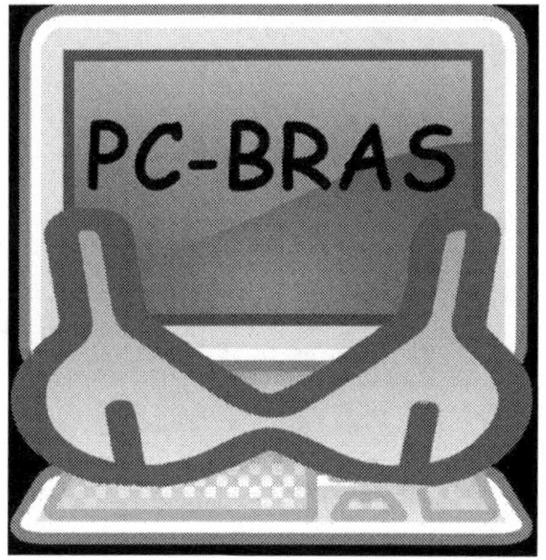

Phenytoin
Carbamazepine

Barbiturates
Rifampicin
Alcohol (chronic use)
Sulphonylureas

Thrombolytic Agents USA:

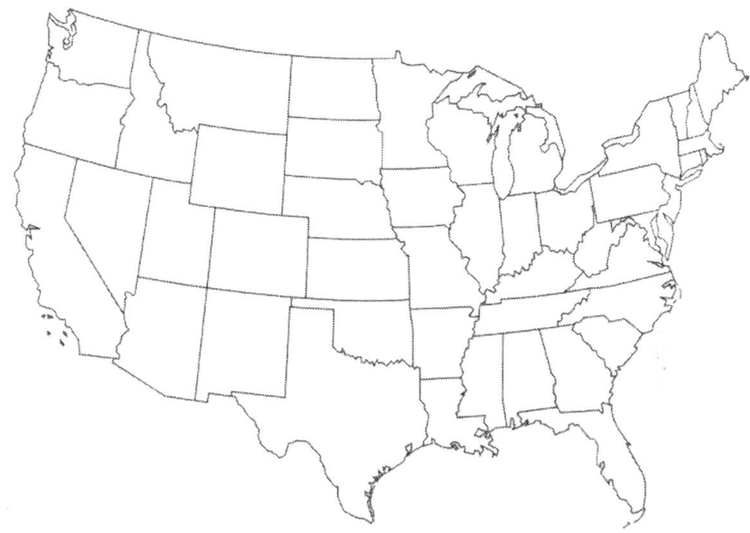

Urokinase **S**treptokinase **A**lteplase (tPA)

Enoxaparin (prototype low molecular weight heparin): action, monitoring EnoXaprin only acts on factor Xa. Monitor Xa concentration, rather than APTT.

Warfarin: Action, Monitoring - We PT:

Warfarin works on the **E**xtrinsic pathway and is monitored by **PT**.

Warfarin: Metabolism SLOW:

- Has a slow onset of action.
- A quicK Vitamin K antagonist, though.

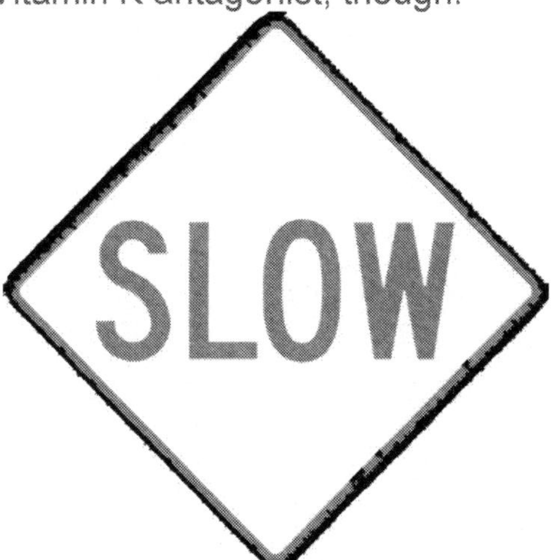

Small lipid-soluble molecule
Liver: site of action
Oral route of administration.
Warfarin

Lead poisoning: presentation ABCDEFG:

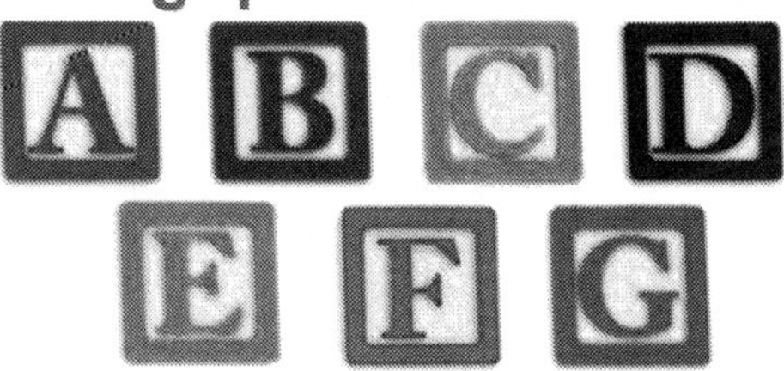

Anemia
Basophilic stripping
Colicky pain
Diarrhea
Encephalopathy
Foot drop
Gum (lead line)

Chapter 11
Neuro

Side Effects Of Sodium Valproate (VALPROATE)

- **V**omiting
- **A**lopecia
- **L**iver toxicity
- **P**ancreatitis/ **P**ancytopenia
- **R**etention of fat (weight gain)
- **O**edema (peripheral)
- **A**norexia
- **T**remor
- **E**nzyme inhibitor

Antimuscarinics: Members, Action

"**I**nhibits **P**arasympathetic **A**nd **S**weat":

I	P	A	S
p	i	t	c
r	r	r	o
a	e	o	p
t	n	p	o
r	z	i	l
o	e	n	a
p	p	e	m
i	i		i
u	n		n
m	e		e

Muscarinic receptors at all parasympathetic endings sweat glands in sympathetic.

CARE Drugs To Treat Alzheimer's

Cognex
Aricept
REminyl
Exelon

Muscarinic effects SLUG BAM:

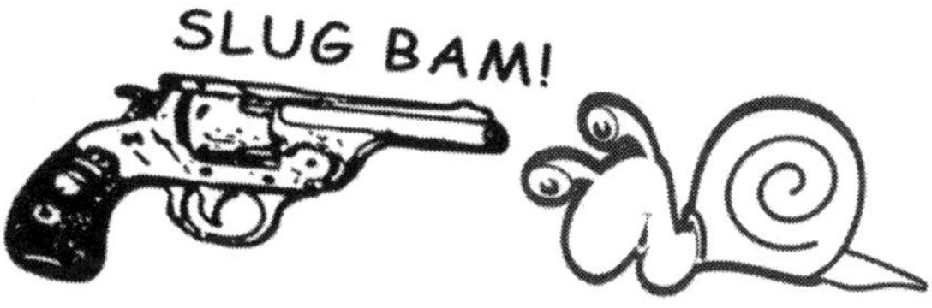

Salivation/ **S**ecretions/ **S**weating
Lacrimation
Urination
Gastrointestinal upset
Bradycardia/ **B**ronchoconstriction/ **B**owel movement
Abdominal cramps/ **A**norexia
Miosis

Cholinergic Crisis: SLUDGE

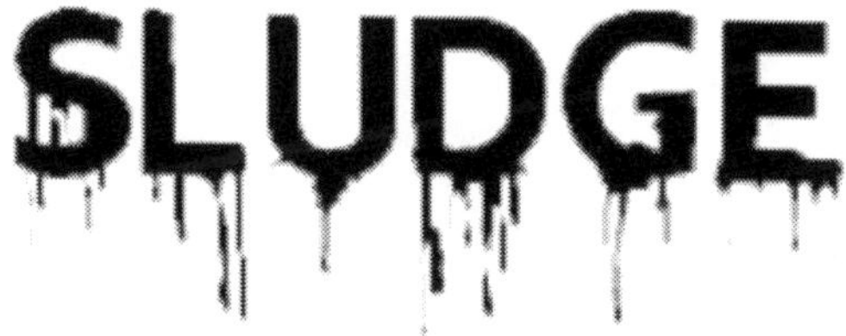

Salvation
Lacrimation
Urination
Defecation
Gastric upset
Emesis

Epilepsy Types, Drugs Of Choice:

"Military General Attacked Weary Fighters Proclaiming 'Veni Vedi Veci' After Crushing Enemies":

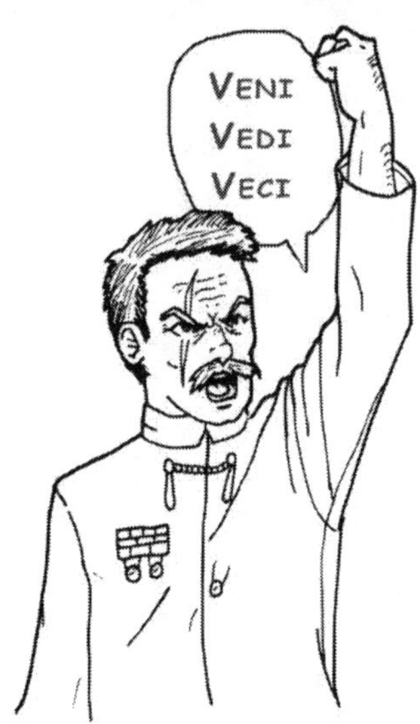

- · Epilepsy types: **M**yoclonic, **G**rand mal, **A**tonic, **W**est syndrome. **F**ocal, **P**etit mal (absence)
- · Respective drugs: **V**alproate **V**alproate **V**alproate **A**CTH **C**arbamazepine **E**thosuximide

Migraine: Prophylaxis Drugs

"Very Volatile Pharmacotherapeutic Agents For Migraine Prophylaxis":

Verapamil
Valproic acid
Pizotifen
Amitriptyline
Flunarizine
Methysergide
Propranolol

Physostigmine vs. Neostigmine LMNOP:

Lipid soluble
Miotic
Natural
Orally absorbed well
Physostigmine

Neostigmine, on the Contrary, Is:

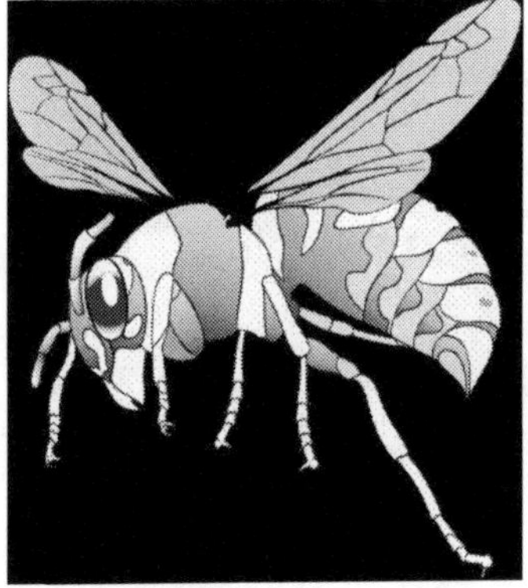

Water soluble
Administered in myasthenia gravis
Synthetic
Poor oral absorption

SIADH-Inducing Drugs ABCD:

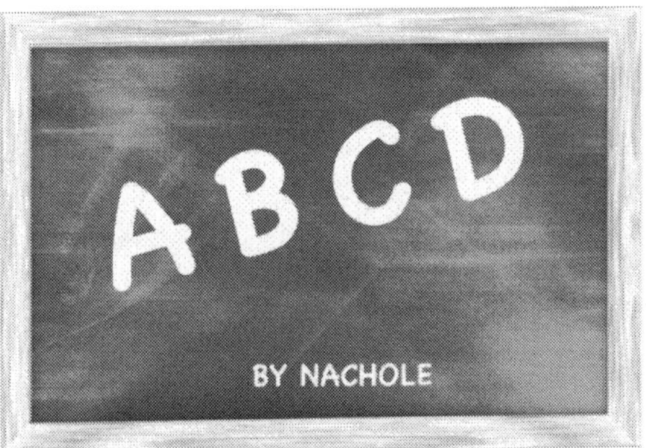

Analgesics: opioids, NSAIDs
Barbiturates
Cyclophosphamide/ **C**hlorpromazine/ **C**arbamazepine
Diuretic (thiazide)

Phenobarbital: Side Effects

Children are annoying

(hyperkinesia, irritability, insomnia, aggression).

Adults are dozy

(sedation, dizziness, drowsiness)

Phenytoin: adverse effects PHENYTOIN:

P-450 interactions
Hirsutism
Enlarged gums
Nystagmus
Yellow-browning of skin
Teratogenicity
Osteomalacia
Interference with B12 metabolism (hence anemia)
Neuropathies: vertigo, ataxia, and headache

Anticholinergic Side Effects

"Know the ABCD'S of anticholinergic side effects":

Anorexia
Blurry vision
Constipation/ **C**onfusion
Dry Mouth
Sedation/ Stasis of urine

Myasthenia Gravis: Edrophonium Vs. Pyridostigmine

e**D**rophonium is for **D**iagnosis.
py**RID**ostigmine is to get **RID** of symptoms.

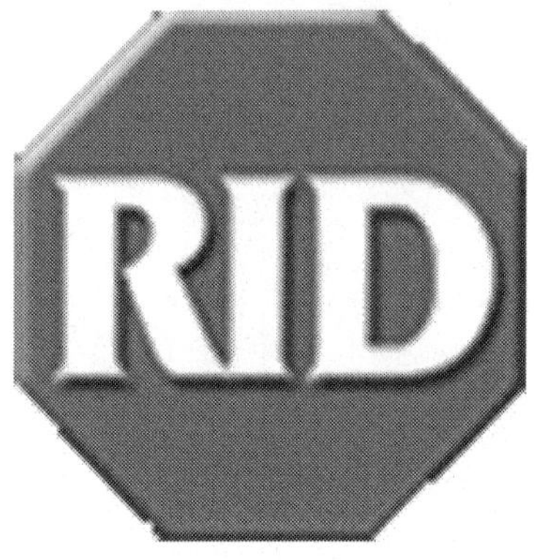

Cholinergics (e.g. Organophosphates): Effects

If you know these, you will be "LESS DUMB":

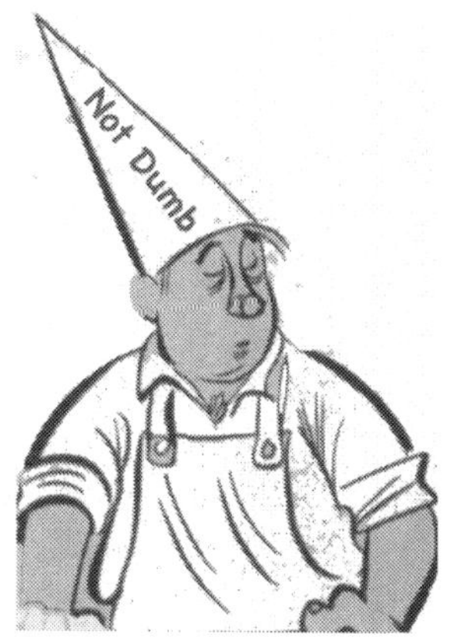

Lacrimation
Excitation of nicotinic synapses
Salivation
Sweating

Diarrhea
Urination
Micturition
Bronchoconstriction

Methyldopa:

Side Effects METHYLDOPA:

Mentally challenged
Electrolyte imbalance
Tolerance
Headache/ **H**epatotoxicity
ps**Y**chological upset
Lactation in women
Dry mouth
Oedema
Parkinsonism
Anemia (hemolytic)

Botulism Toxin: Action, Related Bungarotoxin

Action: "Botulism Bottles up the Ach so it can't be the released":

Related bungarotoxin: "Botulism is related to Beta Bungarotoxin (beta-, not alpha-bungarotoxin--alpha has different mechanism).

Other Books by Nachole Johnson

Medical Mnemonics for the Family Nurse Practitioner
NP School and Beyond: Tips for the Student Nurse Practitioner
The Financially Savvy Nurse Practitioner: Your Guide to Building Wealth
50+ Business Ideas For The Entrepreneurial Nurse
You're a Nurse and Want to Start Your Own Business? The Complete Guide
Adult-Gero and Family Nurse Practitioner Certification Review: Labs For Primary Care
Adult-Gero and Family Nurse Practitioner Certification Review: Mental Health
Adult-Gero and Family Nurse Practitioner Certification Review: Cardiac
Adult-Gero and Family Nurse Practitioner Certification Review: Health Promotion
Adult-Gero and Family Nurse Practitioner Certification Review: Pulmonary
Adult-Gero and Family Nurse Practitioner Certification Review: Genitourinary and STDs
Adult-Gero and Family Nurse Practitioner Certification Review: Neuro
Adult-Gero Primary Care and Family Nurse Practitioner Certification Review: Head, Ears, Eyes, Nose, and Throat

Nachole's Amazon Author Page:
amazon.com/author/nacholejohnson
Nachole's Blog: renursing.com

Made in the USA
Las Vegas, NV
28 November 2023

81738906R00052

www.doctorshangout.com/page/pharmacology-mnemonics

www.medical-institution.com

www.medscape.com/viewarticle/825053#vp_2

www.prep4usmle.com

www.quizlet.com

www.scribd.com

www.wikepedia.com

References

Bentz, P.M. & Ellis, J. R. (2007). *Modules For Basic Nursing Skills* (7th ed.) Philadelphia: Lippincott Williams and Wilkins. p 823

Jarvis. C. (2004). *Math For Nurses: Pocket Guide To Dosage Calculation And Drug Preparation* (18th ed.) Upper Saddle River, NJ. Pearson Education. Inc. pp.573-574

Duell, D. J., Martin, B.C., & Smith, S. F. (2004). *Clinical Nursing Skills: Basic To Advanced Skills* (16th ed.) Upper Saddle River, NJ. Pearson Education. Inc. pp 573-574

Perry, A.G., & Potter, P.A. (2006). *Clinical Nursing Skills And Techniques* (6th ed.). St. Louis, MO: Elsevier Mosby. pp. 618-620

http://www.mudphudder.com/medical-mnemonics/mnemonics-pharmacology-toxicology/

http://www.nursefuel.com/8-important-nursing-concepts-every-nursing-student-must-master/?utm_content=buffer618b5&utm_medium=social&utm_source=pinterest.com&utm_campaign=buffer

http://learningmedications.weebly.com/mnemonics.html

http://www.rxpgonline.com/medicalmnemonic911720.html